I0441623

Anti Inflammatory Diet

Strategies to Eliminate Joint Pain, Improve Your Immune System, and Restore Your Overall Health

Matthew Ward

The information herein is offered for informational purposes solely, and is universal as so. The presentation of the information is without contract or any type of guarantee assurance.

The trademarks that are used are without any consent, and the publication of the trademark is without permission or backing by the trademark owner. All trademarks and brands within this book are for clarifying purposes only and are the owned by the owners themselves, not affiliated with this document.

Disclaimer: This book is for informational purposes only. Use of the guidelines in this book is a choice of the reader. This book is not intended for the treatment or prevention of disease. This book is also, not a substitute for medical treatment or an alternative to medical advice.

Matthew Ward

Table of Contents

Introduction

This book contains proven steps and strategies on how to combat chronic inflammation naturally.

In this book, you'll understand how inflammation works, what chronic inflammation is, what is causing it, and how you can help treat or prevent it through the Anti-Inflammatory Diet. Then, you will find practical strategies on how to implement the Anti-Inflammatory Diet by following a series of concrete steps, including a wide variety of recipes. Discover over forty recipes for breakfast, lunch, dinner, snacks, smoothies, salads, and soups that are suitable to those who want to treat or prevent chronic inflammation.

This book is for all ages who want to start a healthy lifestyle and reduce their risk of developing a wide range of diseases caused by chronic inflammation. It is especially helpful to those who have been suffering from long-term and chronic diseases such as diabetes and osteoarthritis. While this book should never be treated as an alternative to professional treatment, it is nevertheless a perfect complement to any health program you may be following.

Through this book, you will be able to take control of your health and improve your overall quality of life. Get started on the Anti-Inflammatory Diet right now by turning to Chapter 1!

Chapter 1: What is Inflammation?

Everyone, throughout their lifetime, has experienced inflammation in certain parts of their body. It is completely natural and one function, out of many, of the immune system. To explain inflammation, we must first discuss how the immune system works.

The Immune System: Your Personal Bodyguard

The human body is an interesting specimen. It is so complex that modern science can't explain many of its functions. However, one of the mechanisms that have been explored in detail is the **immune system**. It is basically the system in the body that protects it from pathogenic organisms (such as toxins, microbes, and bacteria), parasites, and foreign substances (such as a sliver of wood from a splinter). Its means of protection is producing an immune response, one of which is **inflammation.**

Without the immune system, it would only be a matter of hours before all the pathogens and foreign substances ate away at your cells. This is what happens when you die, actually. As soon as the immune system shuts down, the body becomes "torn down and broken up" until all you are left with is your skeleton. It sounds a bit morbid, but this is just to show you how important it is to keep the immune system strong.

The only time we really notice that something is wrong is when the immune system is unable to do its job properly. Here is an example of a normally functioning immune system versus one that is not functioning well enough

(Warning: this might be a bit graphic, so if you cannot bear it you can skip the following part):

> Scenario: You picked on a hangnail without really paying much attention to it. By doing so, you accidentally cut yourself to the point that the area bled. As soon as this happens, all sorts of pathogens in the air try to enter the opening in your skin.
>
> *If your immune system is functioning normally...*
>
> The affected area would immediately become inflamed to isolate it from the rest of the body and prevent the pathogens from spreading. The blood platelets would start to clot to seal the wound and the white blood cells become concentrated on killing the pathogens that have managed to enter the affected area, thus causing pus.
>
> *If you have a weak immune system...*
>
> The area would get infected and will take a long time to heal.

As you can see, the immune system works fast and methodically. Now, let's take a closer look at all the different components of the immune system:

The Entryway Guards: The Skin and The Mucous Membrane

The Skin. The most visible part of the immune system would have to be the skin. It is your body's "wall" against everything and it is tough and impenetrable to pathogens just as long as it stays healthy. The top layer or the epidermis, for instance, have *Langerhans* cells in it, which act as the immune system's siren, in that it sends a warning to let the body know that it is being attacked.

The skin is also flexible enough to cause it to stretch when inflammation occurs, and to go back to its original form - or close to it – once the inflammation has subsided.

The mucous membrane. This is the lining found in the eyes, nose, mouth, and other parts of the body such as the urinary bladder, lungs, stomach, and intestines. One of its main functions is to produce mucus, which contains *lysozyme*, an enzyme that destroys the cell wall of bacteria that try to enter the body. Anything that isn't immediately destroyed becomes trapped in the mucus anyway, and will be spit out, or swallowed and destroyed by the stomach's strong acids.

If a pathogen does penetrate through these defenses nonetheless, then it still has to go through even more complex attacks from within, as discussed below.

The Internal Immune System

The immune system within your body is even more complex, and they consist of the following (prepare for a mouthful): the lymphatic system, thymus, spleen, bone marrow, antibodies, and the complement system.

Here's how each of them works:

3

Lymphatic system. This is a complex, interconnected system of vessels and spaces that are found in between the organs and tissues of the body. It is through this system that **lymph** circulates. Lymph is the plasma-like fluid that contains the white blood cells and chyle, or a milky fluid that contains emulsified fats. You might think that the lymphatic system is similar to the circulatory system, but the main difference is that it doesn't have a heart that would "pump" it. Rather, it oozes to the lymph nodes through normal muscle movement, kind of like how water is manipulated in a rain gutter.

The main role of the lymph system is to obtain water, oxygen, and nutrients from the blood to the cells in the body. Likewise, the cells create waste products and proteins which are absorbed by the lymph to be excreted out. Moreover, lymph is responsible for detecting and getting rid of any bacteria that infiltrates the body. They bring these to the lymph nodes, which will then become inflamed as it filters out the pathogen. This is why you can tell whether you have an infection when your lymph nodes are swollen.

Thymus. At the base of your neck is a ductless glandular organ that is responsible for excreting lymphocytes.

Spleen. This is a large, deep red, egg-shaped organ that is found on the left side of the upper abdomen, between the diaphragm and stomach. It is responsible for filtering the blood for pathogens and old cells that need to be replaced. Some people have their spleens removed, and as a result, their immune system weakens.

Bone marrow. The cavities of the bones are filled with fatty networks of connective tissue called bone marrow. It is responsible for manufacturing stem cells, the fundamental form of both red and white blood cells.

Antibodies. White blood cells produce antibodies, which are also called gamma globulins and immunoglobulin. These antibodies are responsible for detecting specific bacteria, toxins, or viruses called antigen. They then bind to the antigen and disable its damaging effects on the body.

Complement system. This is a group of proteins that are found in the blood and created in the liver. Their role is to complement or support the antibodies by triggering cells to burst and signal phagocytes that a certain cell needs to be taken out.

Completely, a healthy immune system is necessary to protect our body from infection. However, it becomes a life-threatening problem when the immune system malfunctions, leading to **chronic inflammation**. Unfortunately, many people are unaware of its dangers. What is worse, is they continue to eat food that only aggravate this malfunction. Learn more about it in the next chapter.

Chapter 2: Why and How Does Inflammation Occur?

As discussed in the previous chapter, inflammation is a natural, healthy immune response, of the body, to threats. When a part of your body becomes inflamed, painful, red, and hot, it is your body telling you that something is wrong with it. This also indicates that your immune systems is doing the best it can to fix the matter.

However, when the immune system is constantly triggered to go on defense, then chronic inflammation occurs, causing you to become susceptible to many diseases. Chronic inflammation is when the body is continuously exposed to irritation. In rare cases, it is the immune system itself that attacks its own cells, a condition classified as an autoimmune disease. However, for the most part, chronic inflammation can be treated or avoided once you have identified and eliminated what the root cause is.

Diseases Linked to Chronic Inflammation

The problem with chronic inflammation is that you wouldn't be able to detect it. However, chronic inflammation can manifest in the form of other diseases. Here is a list of the diseases as well as their symptoms that you need to look out for:

Allergies

Those who have persistent acne or other skin conditions are likely to be eating some food, or exposed to certain substances, that cause allergy. In addition, there are other symptoms such as stomach pain, other digestive issues, itchy and watery eyes, runny nose, and chronic lethargy.

Inflammatory Bowel Disease

If your bowels are inflamed, you are likely to find blood or mucus in your stools and you often experience diarrhea or constipation. Because of these symptoms, your appetite decreases, leading to poor food intake and subsequently chronic fatigue.

Rheumatoid Arthritis or Osteoarthritis

Joint pain and inflammation are the obvious symptoms of this disease, as well as weakness and weight loss.

Multiple Sclerosis

Sclerosis is a pathological hardening of the tissue, and its symptoms are often associated with a tingling sensation or weakness in the area. Blurred vision and dizziness also accompany these symptoms.

Diabetes

This disease has many symptoms, but often the person would experience an increase in thirst and hunger throughout the day as well as in a frequent desire to urinate.

Heart Disease

Often, cardiovascular disease is asymptomatic, unless it is reflected in your blood pressure levels. Sometimes fatigue, dizziness, and sweating are also experienced but not in everyone.

Celiac Disease

If you have frequent digestive issues such as diarrhea or constipation with greasy stools, you might have this disease.

The Causes of Chronic Inflammation

An increasing number of people are experiencing chronic inflammation because of many factors. Most of them have to do with poor lifestyle choices, which means that you can do something to eliminate chronic inflammation. Here are the main causes:

Poor Diet

Those who regularly eat foods that are processed or high in sodium, sugar, and other additives are more likely to develop chronic inflammation. Fortunately, diet is one of the factors that are under our control when it comes to treating or preventing chronic inflammation.

Chronic Stress

Stress is a natural reaction to anything that the mind perceives as a threat to your life, such as a wild animal that is about to attack you. When the mind is stressed, the body releases specific chemicals, such as adrenaline and cortisol, to trigger you to make quick decisions and move fast enough so as to defend yourself or escape from the threat. Therefore, these hormones temporarily trigger an increase in your heart rate and muscle tension.

However, when the mind is constantly stressed, the body has no choice but to release these chemicals. Even stressors such as an overly demanding job, which is not necessarily life threatening, still trigger these responses. And the more often these chemicals are released into your bloodstream, the more likely it is for your body to attack itself and trigger an immune response. All these lead to chronic inflammation.

Environmental Toxins

Toxins are foreign substances that irritate the body and trigger the immune system to respond through inflammation. This means that if one is constantly exposed to toxic chemicals, he or she is highly likely to experience chronic inflammation as well. Inhaling polluted air, using body products containing toxins, and storing food and beverages in containers that have Bisphenol A (or BPA) are some of the most common causes.

Chronic Infection

Chronic infection can sometimes go undetected for years until it starts to become strong enough to manifest physical symptoms, such as Hepatitis C. Sometimes, chronic inflammation leads to chronic infection, if not the other way around. A weakened immune system leads to chronic infection and is further aggravated by bad habits, such as chain smoking and alcohol addiction.

Allergens

Any substance that triggers an immune response is called an allergen. Even if something is considered as harmless, such as pollen and gluten, the body might still detect it as an allergen, and therefore leads to inflammation. Genetics often play a role on what causes you to have an allergic reaction to certain substances, although further research is needed to support this.

Other causes of chronic inflammation are genetics and dependency on certain medications. However, it's apparent that most of these culprits can actually be avoided.

Poor diet, for instance, is one of the easiest problems to overcome and this book is all about this particular solution. Chronic stress can be avoided through stress management techniques and lifestyle change.

Those who live in an area that constantly exposes them to environmental toxins, particularly in the urban area, should highly consider taking steps towards relocating. Through these changes, you are likely to reduce the frequency of experiencing infection and allergies as your immune system develops.

But going back to the subject of diet, you can learn more about the foods that trigger inflammation and those that help alleviate it in the next chapter.

Chapter 3: Inflammation and Dietary Triggers

Everything that you eat, or drink, each day has a direct impact on your body. In fact, certain foods are known to directly trigger inflammation. There are also foods that help inhibit chronic inflammation.

Foods that Trigger Inflammation

Certain food are known to trigger inflammation, so you must cut them out of your diet especially if you are at high risk of chronic inflammation. Here is a list of the foods you should avoid:

Refined Sugar and Artificial Sweeteners

There is no way around it: sugar is the primary cause of inflammation. Refined sugars are rich in calories, but don't provide any nutrients whatsoever. Yet, people add it in beverages and all sorts of foods, even foods that don't really need the sweetness factor.

Eating too much refined sugar leads to chronic inflammation, obesity, and really bad cavities. It is known for causing insulin levels, in the blood, to spike sky high, which would also leads to developing an increased risk of Type 2 diabetes.

Artificial sweeteners are also just as bad because they contain ingredients such as sucralose, which has been scientifically proven to damage DNA. It's also known for inhibiting the growth of healthy bacteria in the gut, which leads to inflammatory bowel disease and a higher risk of allergies.

If you want to start the habit of cutting our refined sugar and artificial sweeteners from your diet, you begin by avoiding: soft drinks, both regular and diet, cakes, candy, and pastries, corn syrup, sorghum syrup, and golden syrup. Instead, drink more water and unsweetened beverages. If you are craving for something sweet, then munch on some fruit, which happens to be high in nutrients.

Moldy Food

Anything with molds in them can trigger an inflammatory reaction because the body perceives mold as a threat. It may not manifest outwardly (or on your skin) but it may wreak havoc in your digestive tract. So, toss out anything with molds.

Alcoholic beverages

The high acid content in alcohol may cause your throat and digestive tract to become inflamed. Moreover, alcoholic beverages contain yeast, which can irritate your digestive tract.

Commercial, Processed Meat

Processed meat is high in sodium and other chemical additives that can easily trigger inflammation and irritation.

Hydrogenated Oils

Hydrogenated oils are processed to the point where they no longer contain any nutrients. They are high in omega-6 fatty acids which are known to cause high blood cholesterol and inflammation.

Milk and Cheese

Over half, the population is unable to digest dairy, a condition known as lactose intolerance. This triggers stomach pain, acne, and constipation or diarrhea.

As you might have noticed, most dairy foods are in the form of processed food. Keep in mind that certain foods can trigger inflammation to some people and not to others. To know which ones, in particular, you should avoid and which ones you should just eat less of, you can keep a food diary. That way, you can monitor your body's reaction to certain foods as you gradually eliminate each of these from the list.

Here is a list of food that are known to commonly trigger an allergic response:

- Food containing gluten, such as flour, beer, bread, cakes, cereal, cookies, pasta, soy sauce, and deli meats.

- Dairy products, including butter, cheese, cream cheese, and ice cream.

- Corn ad corn products, including corn flour, cornmeal, cornstarch, corn syrup and sugar, corn oil, golden syrup, xanthan gum, maltose, and maltodextrin.

- Soy products, including soy flour, bean curd, miso, soy milk, soy oil, soy protein, tamari, tempeh, tofu, and textured vegetable protein or TVP

- Peanuts

- Caffeinated beverages and food

- Alcohol

- Conventional animal products from industrial farms

- Eggs

- Nightshade vegetables

It is important to remember that you do not have to avoid these foods if you don't have an allergic reaction to them. The reason why some of these foods, such as the nightshade vegetables and eggs, are still present in the recipes in the Anti-Inflammatory Diet, is because they are nevertheless nutritious.

Foods in the Anti-Inflammatory Diet

When food is consumed in its natural state or is minimally processed (such as in the case of steaming and grilling, both of which are meant to increase flavor and kill any bacteria lurking in the food), the digestive system is better able to process it and collect its nutrients.

Fresh Vegetables

Nutritionists recommend that people should eat three servings of vegetables each day. This is why at least half the ingredients in the Anti-Inflammatory Diet consist of them. Vegetables are rich in vitamins, minerals, and other essential nutrients that bolster the immune system's ability to fight off pathogens and promote healing.

Whole or Gluten-Free Grains

Whole grains such as whole wheat, gluten-free grains such as brown rice are tasty, filling, and full of energy and fiber. The nutrients in them, such as manganese and iron, are necessary to promote healthy bones and joints.

Nuts and Some Seeds

Nuts such as almonds, walnuts, pistachios, and seeds such as sunflower seeds and chia seeds are rich in lean protein and omega-3 fatty acids, which are necessary to promote a healthy nervous system.

Beans and Legumes

Beans such as kidney beans and chickpeas, and legumes such as lentils, beans, and peas, are high in complex carbohydrates and lean protein. These are necessary to promote healthy bodily functions and tissue repair.

Probiotic Food

Probiotics are the "good" bacteria that are found in the intestinal tract. They act as a protective layer against the invasive "bad" bacteria. They help prevent inflammation in the digestive tract, therefore reducing your risk of experiencing irritable bowel syndrome and diarrhea. By eating probiotic food such as kimchi, sauerkraut, and yogurt, you are promoting the growth of this healthy bacteria.

Fish Oil and Cold-pressed, Unrefined Oils

Fats might have earned a bad reputation, but in truth, they are necessary because certain vitamins can only be absorbed by the body when consumed along with fats. However, you only need a little bit to reap this benefit, and the best source of healthy fats are from fatty fish such as salmon, mackerel, and sardines, and from cold-pressed, unrefined oils, such as olive oil, avocado oil, sesame seeds oil, and coconut oil.

Natural Sweeteners

Artificial sweeteners and refined sugars should be avoided in order to prevent or treat chronic inflammation, but many people still need a bit of sweetness in their diet. So, to acquire this taste without triggering inflammation, you can turn to natural sweeteners such as pure maple syrup, raw honey, and coconut sugar. Honey, in particular, has anti-bacterial properties that can help soothe inflammation. Just make sure to not consume too much of it because it's still high in sugar.

The only exception, in the Anti-Inflammatory diet, would be natural whole foods that you are allergic to. For instance, whole grains such as brown rice might be considered as natural, but some people are sensitive or even intolerant to them. Others also experience inflammation when they are consuming nightshade fruits and vegetables such as tomatoes, peppers, and eggplant, which means that they should avoid them. This is why it's important to keep a food journal so you know which foods cause your inflammation.

All the same, you should strive to eat meals that are made up of whole foods, preferably locally produced and in season. This might sound tedious at first, but you would be surprised at how much easier, not to mention cheaper and more sustainable, it is to eat clean. In the succeeding chapters, you will learn more about the Anti-Inflammatory Diet and how you can incorporate it into your lifestyle.

Anti-Inflammatory Superfoods

Certain foods have been observed to aid in alleviating the symptoms of chronic inflammation. Make sure to include them into your diet each day so that you can bolster your efforts to overcoming this inflammation. Here is the list of anti-inflammatory superfoods:

Dark Leafy Greens

Spinach, kale, and other dark leafy green vegetables contain anti-inflammatory nutrients, such as vitamins A, B, C, E and K, all of which help reduce cellular damage caused by inflammation.

Basil

Basil contains an enzyme called *eugenol*, which helps alleviate inflammation-causing enzymes.

Apple Cider Vinegar

This natural source of probiotics helps improve the acid levels in the stomach. It's in fact used to help treat many diseases caused by chronic inflammation, including colitis, Crohn's disease, and flu. Make sure to use only raw, unpasteurized apple cider vinegar.

Organic Berries

Berries, especially blueberries, strawberries, blackberries, cranberries, and raspberries, are rich in antioxidants which help reduce inflammation and protect the cells from damage. They are also rich in fiber.

Allium Vegetables

Allium vegetables are garlic, onion, green onion, shallots, leeks, and chives. These help reduce inflammation by helping the immune system combat the triggers with their antibacterial and antiviral compounds.

Fennel

The anti-inflammatory properties of this vegetable are mainly due to *anethole*. It is a substance that helps inhibit the immune system from causing excessive inflammation.

Ginger

Ginger is a superfood that is used to treat many types of illnesses, including arthritis, colds, and digestive issues. A compound named *gingerols*, in particular, helps reduce inflammation.

Dill

This herb helps treat indigestion, bloating, and constipation. It also has anti-cancer and anti-inflammatory properties.

Turmeric

Turmeric is one of the leading superfoods that is known specifically for reducing inflammation. It is the only food that contains *curcumin,* a component that reduces inflammation in the digestive tract and helps boost liver health.

It would be best to keep a list of these anti-inflammatory foods on your refrigerator door, or wherever you can see it, anytime you prepare your meals. That way, you will be reminded of which ingredients to add to each dish.

Chapter 4: What an Anti-Inflammatory Diet Can Do for You

By following the Anti-Inflammatory Diet consistently, you'll be able to reap a wide range of benefits. Some of these benefits will definitely be observable, such as weight loss and higher resistance to illness. However, while the others may not be as observable, they are nevertheless crucial to your overall well-being, such as improved blood pressure and blood sugar levels.

So, without further ado here are some of the benefits that you can get from an Anti-Inflammatory Diet:

Immune System Improvements

By eating food that naturally contain antibacterial, antiviral, and anti-inflammatory properties, your immune system becomes stronger and more resistant to pathogens. Your body's ability to repair damaged tissues and flush out toxins also become more effective.

Decrease or Eliminate Joint Pain

Inflammation and hardening of the tissues, particularly in the joints, is one of the most painful effects of chronic inflammation. This only worsens if you continue to eat foods that trigger further inflammation. However, after you follow the Anti-Inflammatory Diet, you will gradually notice an improvement in the condition of your joints. In time, your body will finally be able to recuperate and heal the damaged tissue in the area and eliminate the pain altogether.

Weight Control Improvements

People who have been following a conventional Western diet (which consists of processed food and does not contain a lot of vegetables) and switched to an anti-inflammatory diet have noticed healthy weight loss. Furthermore, because they have reduced or eliminated saturated and trans fats, sugar, and salt from their diet, they were able to maintain their healthier weight.

Blood Cholesterol Levels Improvements

Aside from weight loss, the Anti-Inflammatory Diet will also greatly improve your cardiovascular health. By eliminating these same inflammation-causing foods, you can help reduce the amount of LDL or the "bad" cholesterol in your blood, which is linked to atherosclerosis and coronary heart disease.

Blood Sugar Stabilization

You'll no longer experience unhealthy spikes and subsequent crashes in terms of energy and mood once you start the anti-inflammatory diet. This is mainly due to the fact that you'll be eating complex carbohydrates (such as brown rice, whole wheat bread, and quinoa), which breaks down slower in the digestive system and therefore releases glucose into the bloodstream slower but steadily. This is the opposite of what simple carbs (such as white flour and refined sugar) do to your body. These cause an immediate rush of glucose in the blood stream, leading to a sudden increase in insulin production which, in time, will force the body to become resistant to insulin and develop Type 2 diabetes.

Decrease Risk of Developing Colon Cancer

It's difficult to point out what the exact cause of colon cancer is, but one of the common reasons is the high consumption of processed food. Chronic inflammation in the digestive tract often goes undetected, and this causes a blockage that leads to further complications. This type of cancer is directly linked to a high fat, low fiber diet, which is what the conventional Western diet is all about. Fortunately, the Anti-Inflammatory Diet is high in fiber and lower in fat, which helps to reduce this risk significantly.

There are plenty of other, often more personal, benefits that you'll notice once you have committed to the Anti-Inflammatory Diet. For instance, those who suffer from acne may notice their skin clearing up. Others who experience hair loss may notice having stronger strands. Others may even experience having improved energy levels to keep them productive throughout the day.

Whatever health concerns, inflammation, you may be experiencing right now, you'll have a better chance of overcoming them when you start to eat healthily and follow the Anti-Inflammatory Diet. But how do you begin? You will find a simple yet concise guide on how to do so in the next chapter.

Chapter 5: The Anti-Inflammatory Strategy

The Anti-Inflammatory Diet is not just a diet, instead, it should be considered a way of life. There is no "deadline" or end goal. Throughout the process, you'll experience all the benefits that are only natural to eating healthy. These include weight loss, lower LDL cholesterol and blood sugar levels, a reduced risk of developing degenerative diseases, and so on.

To successfully replace your current diet with the Anti-Inflammatory Diet, it is important to know specific needs. For instance, you should figure out how many calories you need each day, how much time you can spend on cooking your own food, how often you eat out, which foods are readily available in your area, and so on. By developing a plan that suits your lifestyle, you can turn the Anti-Inflammatory Diet into something that is sustainable and therefore doable for you.

Dietary and Lifestyle Changes

Regardless of how you are going to implement the Anti-Inflammatory Diet, there are specific dietary and lifestyle changes that you should follow. Here is a summary of guidelines you can implement to ensure that you'll reap the full benefits of this diet:

1. Fill half your plate with vegetables and eat them first.

2. Avoid trans fats and saturated fats (specifically processed food and meats) as often as possible.

3. Choose wild-caught fatty fish as your source of lean protein, whenever possible, or munch on walnuts. Skinless chicken is also a better alternative to red meat.

4. Always opt for whole wheat or gluten-free whenever you crave for carbs, such as bulgur wheat or brown rice. Stay away from simple carbs such as white rice, flour, and pasta as often as possible.

5. Snack on nuts, seeds, and fruits (in moderation) instead of packaged food.

6. Use a variety of herbs and spices in your dishes, especially turmeric, basil, dill, garlic, and ginger.

7. Sneak some exercise into your schedule every day. It can be as simple as doing 50 jumping jacks every 3 hours.

8. Follow a consistent, healthy sleeping pattern. Try to go to bed early and wake up early consistently. That way, your meal schedule will also remain regular.

The 66 Day Success Plan to Following the Anti-Inflammatory Diet

The interesting thing about human beings is that, no matter how convincing the facts and figures may be, we still tend to ignore them in favor of what we are used to. For example, we know for a fact that sugar is bad for us, but we continue to add them into our food anyway. This is because we haven't yet developed the right habits to replace the old ones.

So, to ensure that you really are going to follow the Anti-Inflammatory Diet, here are the steps that you need to implement in order to build the right habits:

Step 1: Determine what causes you to eat unhealthy, inflammation-causing foods.

Do you eat processed foods because they are the ones readily available to you? Have you associated certain unhealthy foods to feeling good? Think about healthier alternatives that you can turn to instead of these unhealthy foods whenever you have these cravings.

Step 2: Figure out how you can make anti-inflammatory foods more accessible for you and make inflammation-causing foods difficult to obtain.

Once you have come up with a list of healthier alternatives, make them more available to you. For instance, your kitchen should contain nothing but anti-inflammatory foods.

Step 3: Reward yourself

Encourage yourself to continue eating anti-inflammatory meals. Choose the ones that you enjoy eating the most. Share your progress with your friends on the internet. Do whatever makes you feel good as a reward for following the Anti-Inflammatory Diet (just as long as it does not defeat its own purpose, of course).

With these steps in mind, here is an action plan to help you start this journey:

Days 1 through 22: Start the Anti-Inflammatory Diet. Religiously follow your meal plan, no matter how challenging it may be. Make sure to take note of everything as a reference. It's nice to look back at your progress!

If necessary, you can ask for professional help from a dietitian or nutritionist during this period.

Days 22 to 44: Study your progress from the last 22 days and reflect on how you can make improvements to your diet plan. Adjust your plan according to the notes so that your cooking and eating habits will be more suited to your lifestyle.

Day 44 to 66: Stick to your diet plan no matter what. Stay motivated by reading this book once more and by doing further research on the benefits of the anti-inflammatory foods. Incorporate a little bit of fun to your routine, perhaps by following new recipes or eating out at a healthy, anti-inflammatory diet friendly restaurant.

On the last day, you can reward yourself for following your Anti-Inflammatory Diet plan. You can get a massage, for example, or buy your favorite workout clothes. It is important to reward yourself because it's both encouraging and motivating.

Now that you know the nature of habits and how you can use this action plan to start the Anti-Inflammatory Diet, you're ready to put everything into action. To do that, you should come up with a 66-day meal plan so that you are certain to eat anti-inflammatory foods every day. You will find a guide as well as a wide variety of anti-inflammatory recipes to try out in the next chapter.

Chapter 6: Anti-Inflammatory Recipes

As explained in the previous chapter, it is always better to develop your own personal meal plan that suits your lifestyle. That way, you're sure to follow it every day. Below is a quick guide to help you create your personal meal plan.

The Meal Plan Strategy

Think about how often you usually eat every day. Do you eat three large meals, or do you prefer to eat five small meals? How often do you eat out, and what are the possibilities of you preparing your own meals at home? All these factors and more will determine the kind of meal plan you create. Follow these simple steps and you are well on your way to incorporating the Anti-Inflammatory Diet into your lifestyle:

Step 1: Decide on how many meals you want to have each day.

The number of meals you eat on Mondays might be different than Saturdays, so you can be as detailed or general as you like. Whatever the case may be, write it down on a sheet of paper.

Here is an example:

Mondays through Fridays: Breakfast, Lunch, Afternoon Snack, and Dinner

Saturdays and Sundays: Brunch, Lunch, Afternoon Snack, Dinner, and Evening Snack

Step 2: Consider how often you can cook meals at home.

Cooking your own meals might sound tedious and time-consuming, but the truth is that it can save you a lot more money, time, and energy than eating out. There are several options for you to choose from, such as making meals ahead of time or choosing easy-to-prepare recipes.

Make sure to choose a method of preparing food that you are sure to stick to. If making meals ahead of time is something that you can't follow no matter what, then find an alternative that will still enable you to cook at home without spending too much time in the kitchen. For example, you can choose to slow cook your meals each day, which simply involves throwing together the ingredients into a slow cooker and then letting it do its job.

Here is an example of a plan that combines making meals ahead of time with eating out:

> Sundays: *eat out for brunch, eat leftover meals from Saturday, make breakfast, lunch, and dinner for Monday, Tuesday, and Wednesday ahead of time*

> Wednesdays: *make breakfast for Thursday, Friday, and Saturday ahead of time*

> Thursday: *eat out for lunch, slow cook for Thursday's dinner and Friday's lunch*

> Friday: *eat slow cooked meal from Thursday, eat out on Friday*

Saturday: *cook breakfast, eat out for lunch, slow cook for Saturday and Sunday dinners*

Once you have decided on your meal plan, you should then create one that will last for 66 days, or 9 weeks and 3 days. Start by filling out your meal plan with specific meals for the first two weeks, then repeat the same steps for every subsequent two weeks. If you like, you could even "rotate" the meal plans in that you simply use the exact same meal plan every three weeks or so. By implementing the 66-day rule, you are sure to build the habit of following the Anti-Inflammatory Diet.

Step 3: Gather your recipes, ingredients, and kitchen tools.

After you have carefully created a personalized Anti-Inflammatory Diet plan, you should then put it into action by gathering all the supplies you need.

For example, if you really want to include slow cooking into your plan, then you certainly need a good quality slow cooker. If you wish to make meals ahead of time, then you'll need appropriate airtight containers and a refrigerator in which to store those meals.

Also, it's important to remember that you should have a list of restaurants that serve healthy food and are acceptable in the Anti-Inflammatory Diet. That way, you won't have to worry about deciding where to go, when eating out.

Once you have your plan and kitchen tools all laid out, you can launch it immediately. To get you started below is a series of anti-inflammatory recipes to choose from.

Breakfast Recipes

Ginger Cinnamon Porridge
Number of Servings: 2

You will need:

- 2 cups water
- 1 cup traditional rolled oats (or gluten-free)
- ½ cup raisins
- 2 Tbsp blackstrap molasses
- 2 Tbsp flaxseeds
- 2 tsp ground ginger
- 1 tsp ground cinnamon
- ½ tsp ground nutmeg

How to Prepare:

Pour the water into a saucepan and stir in the oats, ginger, cinnamon, and nutmeg. Place over medium high flame and bring to a boil.

Once boiling, reduce to a simmer and stir in the raisins. Simmer for about 5 minutes, or until fragrant and thickened.

Turn off the heat and stir in the flaxseeds. Cover and let stand for 3 minutes, then stir in the blackstrap molasses. Ladle into serving bowls and serve right away.

Spiced Porridge
Number of Servings: 6 servings

You will need:

- 6 cups water

- 2 cups steel cut oats

- 2 Tbsp ground cinnamon

- 2 tsp ground cinnamon

- 1 ½ tsp ground coriander

- 1/6 tsp ground nutmeg

- 1/3 tsp ground allspice

- 1/3 tsp ground cardamom

- 1/3 tsp ground ginger

- Maple syrup, to taste

How to Prepare:

Pour the water into a pot and place over medium flame. Bring to a simmer, then stir in the oats.

Once combined, stir in the spices. Simmer for 5 minutes, stirring constantly until the mixture is thoroughly combined.

Ladle into soup bowls and add a drizzle of maple syrup on top. Best served warm. Alternatively, store in mason jars, seal, refrigerate overnight and serve chilled.

Simple Pancakes with Honeyed Raspberries
Number of Servings: 3

You will need:

- 2 organic eggs

- 3 cups fresh raspberries

- ½ cup nut milk, such as almond

- 1/3 cup whole wheat or gluten-free flour

- 1 Tbsp raw honey

- ½ tsp pure vanilla paste or extract

- Optional: ½ Tbsp maple or coconut sugar

- Sea salt

How to Prepare:

Combine the honey, raspberries, and sugar, in a bowl. Mix well, then set aside for half an hour.

After half an hour, beat the eggs in a bowl, then mix in the vanilla and milk. Gently stir in the flour with a pinch of salt. Mix well.

Place a cast-iron skillet over medium-low flame and heat through. Ladle in a quarter cup of the batter, then cook for about 30 seconds per side, or until firm. Transfer to a plate and cook the remaining batter the same way. Once the pancakes are ready, spoon the raspberry mixture on top and serve right away.

Zesty Quinoa and Chia Bowl

Number of Servings: 4

You will need:

- 1 cup almond milk

- 1 ½ cups water

- ¾ cup quinoa, rinsed thoroughly

- 3 Tbsp pure maple syrup

- 2 Tbsp slivered almonds

- ¾ Tbsp chia seeds

- 1/8 tsp freshly grated lemon zest

- Sea salt, to taste

How to Prepare:

Boil the water in a pot, then stir in the quinoa and cover.

Simmer over low flame for 15 minutes or until the quinoa is tender and has almost completely absorbed the water. Keep covered for 5 minutes, then drain excess water and set aside.

Stir in the almond milk, maple syrup, chia seeds, lemon zest, salt, and almonds. Mix well, then serve right away.

Korean Breakfast Bibimbap
Number of Servings: 3

You will need:

- 3 eggs, poached
- 1 small carrot, peeled and julienned
- 1 small zucchini, julienned
- 2 green onions, white and light green parts, chopped
- 1 small garlic clove, minced
- 1 ½ cups cooked quinoa or brown rice
- 1 ½ cups sliced shiitake or cremini mushrooms
- ¾ Tbsp chopped fresh mint
- ¾ Tbsp chopped fresh basil
- 3 tsp toasted sesame oil
- ¾ tsp toasted sesame seeds
- Sea salt, to taste

How to Prepare:

Place a nonstick skillet over medium high flame and let it preheat. Once hot, add ¾ teaspoon of sesame oil and swirl to coat.

Add the carrot, green onion, and zucchini, then stir fry until tender. Season to taste with a bit of salt, then set aside.

Reheat the skillet over medium high flame and add another ¾ teaspoon of oil. Swirl to coat, then stir in the mushrooms. Spread out into a single layer, then cook for 3 minutes, until tender.

Stir in the garlic, then sauté until browned. Transfer to a bowl and set aside.

Reheat the skillet over medium high flame and add the remaining sesame oil. Swirl to coat, then sauté the cooked brown rice or quinoa until crisp tender.

Divide the rice or quinoa among three bowls, then top with the vegetables and fresh herbs. Add the poached egg on top of each serving, then top with sesame seeds and serve right away.

Buckwheat and Quinoa Granola

Number of Servings: 9

You will need:

- 1 ½ cups cooked quinoa

- 1 ½ cups buckwheat groats

- ¾ cup traditional rolled oats (gluten-free)

- ¾ cup unsweetened berries, any kind

- 4 ½ Tbsp raw honey

- 4 ½ Tbsp cold-pressed coconut oil

- 1 ½ tsp pure vanilla paste or extract

- 1/3 tsp ground cinnamon

- 1/3 tsp ground ginger

How to Prepare:

Set the oven to 325 degrees F to preheat. Line a baking sheet with parchment paper and set aside.

In a large mixing bowl, combine the coconut oil, raw honey, cinnamon, ginger, and vanilla.

Add the oats, quinoa, and buckwheat groats, then mix well until thoroughly combined.

Transfer the mixture to the prepared baking sheet (you might need two) and spread out well. Bake for about 45 minutes, or until golden brown and crisp.

Carefully take the baking sheet of granola out of the oven and stir in the berries. Set aside to cool completely, then transfer to an airtight container. Best served with nut milk.

Lunch Recipes

Lentil, Fish and Mustard Greens Stew
Number of Servings: 3

You will need:

- 1 medium onion, chopped

- 1 garlic clove, minced

- ½ lb diced white fish fillet

- ½ lb sweet potatoes, peeled and diced

- 3 cups chicken broth

- 3 cups mustard greens (or kale)

- ¾ cup dried lentils

- ¾ Tbsp olive oil

- Sea salt and freshly ground black pepper, to taste

How to Prepare:

Place a pot over medium high flame and heat through. Once hot, add the olive oil and swirl to coat. Add the white fish and cook for 8 minutes or until cooked through.

Stir in the onions and sauté until tender, then add the garlic and sauté until fragrant.

Pour in the broth, then add the sweet potatoes, lentils, and mustard greens. Bring to a boil, then reduce to a simmer. Cover loosely and simmer for 30 minutes or until the lentils are tender.

Season to taste with salt and pepper, then serve right away.

Grilled Mackerel and Mango Tacos
Number of Servings: 4

You will need:

- ½ lb mackerel fillets
- 2 mangoes
- 2 Tbsp chopped fresh cilantro
- 2 Tbsp freshly squeezed lime juice
- 1 Tbsp canola oil
- 1 Tbsp cold-pressed coconut oil
- ¾ tsp sea salt
- ½ tsp chili powder
- ¼ tsp crushed red pepper
- ¼ tsp garlic powder
- ¼ tsp ground cumin

- 1/8 tsp ground oregano

- 4 whole wheat or gluten-free tortillas

How to Prepare:

Place the mackerel fillets in a bowl and add cold water until covered. Set aside for 2 minutes, then drain and blot dry with paper towels. Transfer to a deep dish and set aside.

Combine the canola oil and coconut oil, lime juice, and ½ teaspoon of salt. Add the spices, then mix well. Pour on top of the fish and turn the fish to coat. Cover the dish and marinate for 1 hour.

Peel and dice the mangoes, then place in a bowl. Add the remaining salt and the cilantro, then mix gently. Cover and refrigerate until ready to serve.

To cook the fish, set the grill over medium high heat. Lay the fish on the grill and cook for 3 minutes per side, or until completely cooked. Warm the tortillas on the grill for about 12 seconds per side.

Transfer the grilled fillets to a plate and shred. Spoon into the warmed tortillas, then top with the mango. Serve right away.

Black Bean, Mango and Avocado Burritos
Number of Servings: 3

You will need:

- 1 small red onion, minced

- 1 small mango, peeled, seeded and diced

- 1 small avocado, pitted, peeled and diced

- 3 cups cooked black beans, drained thoroughly

- 2 ½ Tbsp minced fresh cilantro

- 2 Tbsp canola oil

- ¾ Tbsp minced garlic

- 1 ½ tsp minced jalapeno peppers

- 1 ½ tsp freshly squeezed lime juice

- 3 whole wheat tortillas

How to Prepare:

Place a skillet over medium flame and add the canola oil. Swirl to coat, then sauté the red onion, jalapeno pepper, and garlic. Sauté until tender. Add the black beans and sauté for 3 minutes.

Meanwhile, combine the avocado, mango, and cilantro in a bowl. Add the lime juice and toss well to combine.

Warm the tortillas in a toaster oven or dry skillet. Stuff with the black bean mixture, then top with the avocado and mango mixture. Serve right away.

Savory Rice Stuffed Bell Peppers

Number of Servings: 6

You will need:

- 6 large red bell peppers
- 4 green onions, chopped
- 2 celery stalks, chopped
- 32 oz canned crushed tomatoes
- 3 cups diced mushrooms
- 3 cups vegetable broth
- 1 ½ cups uncooked brown rice
- 1 ¼ cups toasted and chopped pecans
- 3 Tbsp olive oil
- 1 ½ Tbsp dried oregano
- 3 tsp dried basil
- 1/3 tsp ground cayenne pepper
- Sea salt and freshly ground black pepper, to taste

How to Prepare:

Set the oven to 350 degrees F to preheat.

Slice the tops off the bell peppers and set aside, then scoop out the seeds. Set them aside.

Place a saucepan over medium high flame and heat through. Once hot, add the olive oil and swirl to coat. Sauté the mushrooms until tender, then stir in the celery, scallions, and brown rice.

Sauté for 4 minutes, then pour in the vegetable broth and stir well to combine. Season with a bit of salt and pepper, then cover and place over a high flame. Bring to a boil, then reduce to a simmer.

Simmer for 45 minutes, or until the rice is puffed and tender.

In the meantime, combine the crushed tomatoes with the cayenne pepper, basil, and oregano in a saucepan. Place over medium high flame and bring to a boil, then reduce to low flame and simmer for 3 minutes or until heated through.

Pour half the tomato mixture into a baking dish, spreading out to cover the bottom. Set aside.

Transfer the cooked brown rice mixture into a bowl, then fold in the pecans. Stuff the bell peppers with the brown rice mixture, then arrange them in the baking dish over the tomato mixture.

Place the tops of the bell peppers on top of them to cover, then pour the remaining tomato sauce on top.

Bake for 30 minutes, or until the bell peppers are tender and heated through. Set on a cooling rack and let stand for 3 minutes. Best served warm.

Fish Curry on Brown Rice
Number of Servings: 3

You will need:

- 3 fish fillets, any kind, 5 oz each
- 2 small tomatoes, diced
- 1 yellow onion, sliced thinly
- 1 bell pepper, any kind, seeded and sliced thinly
- 2 cups water
- 1 cup uncooked brown rice
- 2 ½ Tbsp hot water
- 1 ½ Tbsp canola oil
- ¾ Tbsp curry powder
- 1/3 tsp ground cumin
- 1/3 tsp ground coriander
- 1/3 tsp cayenne pepper
- 1/6 tsp ground turmeric

How to Prepare:

Pour the brown rice into a pot and add 2 cups of water. Cover and place over a high flame. Bring to a boil, then reduce to medium low flame and simmer for 15 to 20 minutes, or until the rice is tender and has absorbed all the water. Set aside.

Meanwhile, place a skillet over medium high flame and heat through. Once hot, add the canola oil and swirl to coat.

Sauté the onion until translucent, then stir in the bell pepper and spices. Sauté for 2 minutes

Lay the fish fillets on top of the mixture, then spoon some of the bell pepper and onion on top. Add the hot water and tomatoes, then cover and bring to a boil. Once boiling, reduce to medium flame and simmer for 10 minutes, or until the fish is cooked through.

Divide the rice among three plates, then lay the fish fillets on top of each serving. Spoon the curry sauce on top, then serve right away.

Chili Tomato Gazpacho
Number of Servings: 3

You will need:

- 2 ½ lb chopped heirloom tomatoes
- ½ cucumber, diced
- 1 red bell pepper, seeded and diced
- 1 red onion, minced
- 1 large celery stalk, diced
- ½ cup diced tomatoes, juices reserved
- ¼ cup diced jicama
- 2 ½ Tbsp apple cider vinegar
- 2 Tbsp chopped fresh parsley
- 2 Tbsp ice water
- 1 Tbsp cold-pressed olive oil
- ½ Tbsp chopped fresh cilantro
- 1 tsp vegetarian Worcestershire sauce
- 1 tsp sea salt
- 1 tsp ground coriander
- ¾ tsp green Tabasco sauce
- ½ tsp ground cumin

- ¼ tsp ground cayenne

How to Prepare:

Combine all the ingredients in a bowl. Mix well, then pour three-quarters of the mixture into a high powder blender. Blend until smooth, then pour back into the bowl and stir well.

Cover the bowl and refrigerate for at least 1 hour or until chilled. Best served cold with some whole wheat or gluten-free bread.

Dinner Recipes

Baked Lemon Halibut with Spicy Tomato Salsa
Number of Servings: 4

You will need:

- 4 halibut steaks, 6 oz each

- 2 fennel bulbs, sliced

- ½ cup water

- 1 Tbsp crushed black peppercorns

For the Marinade:

- 1/3 cup chopped fresh cilantro

- 2 Tbsp freshly squeezed lemon juice

- ¾ Tbsp freshly grated lemon zest

- ¾ Tbsp cold-pressed olive oil

- ¾ Tbsp freshly grated ginger

- ½ tsp freshly ground black pepper

For the Spicy Tomato Salsa:

- 1 cup diced fresh tomatoes, juices reserved
- 1 small red bell pepper, seeded and diced
- 1 small red onion, diced
- ½ jalapeno pepper, minced
- 1/3 cup chopped fresh cilantro
- 1 ½ Tbsp freshly squeezed lime juice

How to Prepare:

In a nonreactive bowl, combine all the ingredients for the tomato salsa and mix well. Cover and refrigerate until ready to serve.

In a large baking dish, combine all the ingredients for the marinade. Mix well, then add the halibut steaks and turn several times to coat. Cover the dish and refrigerate for at least 2 hours to marinate.

After marinating, set the oven to 400 degrees F to preheat.

Meanwhile, boil just a half cup of water in a saucepan and add the fennel. Simmer, covered, for 7 minutes or until tender. Drain and set aside.

Lay the halibut steaks on a baking dish and pour the marinade on top. Top with peppercorns, then bake for 5 minutes, then turn them over and bake for an added 5 minutes.

Divide the steamed fennel among four plates, then lay one baked halibut over each bed of fennel. Spoon the spicy tomato salsa on top, then serve right away.

Baked Salmon and Zucchini

Number of Servings: 6

You will need:

- 6 salmon fillets, 5 oz each
- 6 zucchinis, chopped
- 3 garlic cloves, minced
- 3 Tbsp chopped fresh parsley
- 3 Tbsp brown sugar
- 3 Tbsp olive oil
- 3 Tbsp freshly squeezed lemon juice
- 1 ½ Tbsp Dijon mustard
- ¾ tsp dried dill
- 1/3 tsp dried oregano
- 1/3 tsp dried rosemary
- Sea salt and freshly ground black pepper, to taste

How to Prepare:

Set the oven to 400 degrees F to preheat. Line a baking sheet with parchment paper and set aside.

Combine the thyme, rosemary, dill, oregano, garlic, lemon juice, Dijon mustard, and brown sugar. Add a pinch of salt and pepper, then mix well and set aside.

Spread the zucchini on the prepared baking sheet then add some olive oil. Season lightly with salt and pepper, then toss to coat.

Lay the salmon fillets on top of the zucchini, then lightly rub the herb mixture on both sides.

Bake for 15 minutes, or until cooked through.

Transfer to a serving dish, then top with parsley and serve right away.

Tuna Steak with Strawberry Walnut Sauce
Number of Servings: 2

You will need:

- 2 fresh tuna steaks, 5 oz each

- 4 oz fresh green beans, trimmed

- ½ lb mixed baby greens, rinsed thoroughly

- ¼ cup almond slivers

- ½ lemon, halved

- Sea salt, to taste

- Freshly ground black pepper, to taste

- Canola oil spray

For the Sauce:

- 1 cup fresh strawberries

- ¼ cup walnuts

- 1 Tbsp cold-pressed walnut or extra virgin olive oil

- 1 Tbsp apple cider vinegar

- ½ Tbsp freshly squeezed lemon juice

- ½ Tbsp Dijon mustard

- ½ Tbsp minced fresh mint leaves

- Freshly ground black pepper, to taste

How to Prepare:

Pour all the ingredients for the sauce in a food processor or blender. Blend until smooth, then pour into a bowl and refrigerate until ready to serve.

Preheat the grill to medium high.

Lightly coat the tuna steaks with canola oil spray. Season lightly with salt and pepper. Grill the tuna for 5 minutes per side, turning only once.

Meanwhile, steam the green beans until crisp tender, then plunge into ice water. Drain and set aside.

Divide the mixed baby greens between two plates, then lay the green beans on top. Add the grilled tuna, then spoon the strawberry walnut sauce on top. Garnish with almonds and lemon wedges, then serve right away.

Hearty Beef Stew
Number of Servings: 4

You will need:

- 1 lb boneless beef top sirloin, sliced into cubes
- 9 oz new potatoes, halved
- 1 large garlic clove, minced
- 2 cups beef broth
- ¾ cup diced carrot
- ¾ cup diced yellow onion
- ¾ cup diced celery
- 3 Tbsp olive oil
- 2 ½ Tbsp tomato paste
- 2 Tbsp brown rice flour
- 1 ½ Tbsp freshly squeezed lemon juice
- 1 ½ tsp raw honey
- 1/3 tsp sea salt
- Ground allspice, to taste
- Freshly ground black pepper, to taste
- Smoked Spanish paprika, to taste

How to Prepare:

Place a stock pot over medium high flame and heat through. Add 1 ½ tablespoons of olive oil and swirl to coat.

Add the beef cubes and sauté until browned all over, then transfer to a plate and set aside.

Place the new potatoes in a bowl with a few tablespoons of hot water. Loosely cover and microwave for 4 minutes or until tender. Set aside.

Add the remaining oil in the stock pot, then heat over a medium flame. Stir in the onion, steamed potato, carrot, celery, garlic, and salt. Sauté until tender, then stir in paprika, allspice, and black pepper to taste. Sauté until combined.

Add the brown rice flour and sauté for 2 minutes, then pour in the broth and simmer for 1 minute. Stir in the lemon juice, honey, and tomato paste, then add the beef.

Reduce to medium low flame and simmer for 8 minutes, or until the beef is tender and cooked through.

Ladle into soup bowls and serve right away.

Broiled Italian-Style Halibut

Number of Servings: 3

You will need:

- 3 halibut fillets, 6 oz each
- 1 cup grape tomatoes
- 1/3 cup pitted kalamata olives
- 1/3 cup chopped tomatoes
- 3 Tbsp cold-pressed olive oil
- 2 ½ Tbsp minced fresh parsley
- 1 ½ Tbsp chopped fresh basil
- 1 Tbsp capers
- 1 ½ tsp minced garlic
- Olive oil spray

How to Prepare:

Combine the olive oil, basil, and half the garlic in a bowl. Set aside for 15 minutes.

After 15 minutes, coat the halibut fillets with the mixture.

Preheat the broiler.

Lay the fillets on a broiler pan and broil for 3 minutes per side, or until cooked through.

Meanwhile, lightly spritz a skillet with olive oil spray, then place over medium flame. Add the grape tomatoes, olives, and capers. Sauté until the tomatoes are tender. Add the rest of the garlic with the chopped tomatoes, then sauté for 4 minutes.

Once the halibut fillets are cooked, transfer to a serving dish and spoon the tomato mixture on top. Garnish with parsley, then serve right away.

All-Veggie Shepherd's Pie
Number of Servings: 9

You will need:

- 3 sweet potatoes, peeled and sliced
- 9 white potatoes, peeled and sliced
- 2 small zucchinis, sliced
- 3 large garlic cloves
- 5 ½ cups water
- 1 ½ cups chopped onion
- 1 ½ cups chopped shiitake mushrooms
- 1 ½ cups lentils
- ¾ cup chopped broccoli florets
- ¾ cup chopped red bell pepper

- 1 ½ Tbsp cold-pressed olive oil

- 1 ½ Tbsp cornstarch

- 1 ½ Tbsp Cajun seasoning

- 1 ½ Tbsp Italian seasoning

- 1 ½ tsp curry powder

- 1 tsp sea salt

- 2 bay leaves

How to Prepare:

Set the oven to 350 degrees F to preheat.

Boil the water in a pot, then add the sweet potatoes and white potatoes. Boil for about 30 to 45 minutes, or until extra tender. Set aside 3 cups of the water, then drain out the rest into another pot.

Pour the reserved water back into the pot, then mash everything until smooth. Fold in ¾ of the olive oil, 1 ½ teaspoons Cajun seasoning, and the Italian seasoning. Mix well.

Boil the water in the other pot over a high flame. Add more, if needed. Add the bay leaves, lentils, and remaining Cajun seasoning. Simmer for 30 to 45 minutes, or until the lentils are tender.

Meanwhile, place a skillet over a medium flame and heat through. Once hot, add the olive oil and swirl to coat. Sauté the onion and mushrooms until tender, then add the bell pepper, garlic, and broccoli. Add about a cup of water, cover, and simmer until broccoli is almost tender.

Season with the salt and curry powder, then mix well. Add the broccoli mixture to the lentil mixture and stir to combine.

Set aside 1/3 cup of the water in a cup, then stir the cornstarch into it. Add the cornstarch mixture into the lentil and broccoli mixture and stir until thickened. Set aside.

Lay the zucchini slices in a large casserole (or two, if needed). Spread half the mashed potatoes over the zucchini layer, then add the lentil and broccoli mixture on top. Add the remaining mashed potato on top, then spread out until smooth.

Bake for 1 hour, or until golden brown. Set on a cooling rack and let stand for 10 minutes before serving. Extra servings can be refrigerated for up to 3 days or frozen for up to 3 months. Reheat before serving.

Snack Recipes

Coconut Carrot Bites

Number of Servings: 27 (pieces)

You will need:

- 1 large carrot, peeled and grated
- 9 pitted dates
- 3 cups chopped cashews
- 1 ¼ cups rolled oats
- ½ cup unsweetened shredded coconut
- 1/3 cup protein powder
- 1/3 cup unsweetened applesauce
- 1/3 cup chopped pecans
- 1/3 cup chopped walnuts
- ¾ tsp ground cinnamon
- 1/6 tsp ground ginger
- 1/3 tsp ground nutmeg

How to Prepare:

67

Combine the spices with the protein powder, oats, spices, dates, and applesauce in a food processor or blender. Blend until the mixture becomes thick and doughy.

Pour in the pecans, walnuts, and shredded carrot, then process until thoroughly combined. Set aside.

Pour the shredded coconut into a plate. Using a spoon, scoop some of the dough from the mixture and roll into a ball.

Coat the mixture in the shredded coconut, then arrange on a platter. Cover with plastic wrap and refrigerate for about an hour or until firm and chilled. Best served chilled.

Easy Garlic Hummus

Number of Servings: 4

You will need:

- 2 garlic cloves, peeled

- 1 ½ cups cooked or canned and rinsed chickpeas, drained well

- 3 Tbsp freshly squeezed lemon juice

- 4 tsp cold-pressed extra virgin olive oil

How to Prepare:

Combine the lemon juice, olive oil, garlic, and chickpeas in a food processor. Blend to the desired level of chunkiness or smoothness.

Pour into a container with an airtight lid and refrigerate. Serve chilled with your favorite vegetable sticks, such as celery, carrot, cucumber, jicama, and bell peppers.

Avocado, Black Bean, and Tomato Bowls
Number of Servings: 3

You will need:

- 1 large avocado

- 10 oz canned black beans, rinsed and drained thoroughly

- ½ jalapeno, minced

- 1 ½ cups halved cherry tomatoes

- 1 ½ Tbsp chopped fresh cilantro

- 1 ½ Tbsp minced white onion

- 1 ½ Tbsp freshly squeezed lime juice

- Sea salt, to taste

How to Prepare:

In a bowl, mix together the tomato, onion, cilantro, and half the lime juice. Add the jalapeno and toss gently to coat. Refrigerate until ready to serve.

Place a saucepan over medium flame and heat through. Once hot, add the black beans and remaining lime juice, then stir well until combined. Season to taste with salt, then stir until heated through. Set aside.

Halve the avocado and discard the stone. Scoop out the flesh and place in a bowl. Add a pinch of salt and mash well until smooth.

Divide the avocado into three bowls and divide the black beans on top. Add the tomato mixture, then serve right away.

Savory Stir-fried Brussels Sprouts

Number of Servings: 3

You will need:

- 1 ½ lb Brussels sprouts

- 1 red onion, minced

- 3 Tbsp cold-pressed olive oil

- 1 ½ tsp red pepper flakes

- 1/3 tsp ground nutmeg

- Sea salt, to taste

How to Prepare:

Dice the Brussels sprouts and set aside.

Place a wok or skillet over medium flame and heat through. Once hot, add the olive oil and swirl to coat. Sauté the onion with the red pepper flakes and a pinch of salt. Stir until translucent and slightly browned.

Add the Brussels sprouts and stir fry for about 5 minutes or until bright green and tender. Add the nutmeg and mix well. Turn off the heat and transfer to a plate. Serve right away.

Roasted Eggplant and Walnut Paste

Number of Servings: 4

You will need:

- 1 small eggplant

- 1 garlic clove, peeled

- ½ cup chopped walnuts

- ½ Tbsp cold-pressed extra virgin olive oil

- 1 tsp peeled and diced fresh ginger

- Ground allspice, to taste

- Sea salt, to taste

- Freshly ground black pepper, to taste

How to Prepare:

Set the oven to 450 degrees F to preheat. Pierce the eggplant all over with a fork, then roast for about 30 minutes, or until extra tender.

Meanwhile, pulse the walnuts in a food processor until roughly ground and set aside.

After the eggplant is roasted, set aside to cool. Once cool to the touch, peel and place the flesh into the food processor with the ground walnuts. Add the olive oil, ginger, and garlic, then blend until smooth.

Season to taste with allspice, salt, and pepper and blend again to combine. Transfer to a container with an airtight lid and refrigerate. Serve chilled with your favorite vegetable sticks, such as celery, carrot, cucumber, jicama, and bell peppers.

Chili Green Beans

Number of Servings: 3

You will need:

- 3 cups green beans, chopped into bite-sized pieces
- 4 ½ cups boiling water
- 3 ½ cups ice cold water
- Chili powder, to taste
- Sea salt and freshly ground black pepper, to taste

How to Prepare:

Rinse the green beans thoroughly, then place in a heatproof bowl and add the boiling water. Stir in a pinch of salt, then let stand for 2 minutes.

Drain thoroughly, then transfer the green beans to a bowl of ice cold water to keep them from overcooking.

Transfer the green beans to a colander and allow to drain. Then, transfer to a serving dish and season with salt, pepper, and chili powder. Toss to coat, then serve right away.

Smoothie Recipes

Coconut, Pineapple and Almond Smoothie
Number of Servings: 2

You will need:

- ¾ cup fresh pineapple, sliced

- 2/3 cup frozen or chilled pineapple juice

- 2 ½ Tbsp almonds

- 2 ½ Tbsp coconut milk

- 1/3 tsp pure maple syrup

How to Prepare:

Combine all the ingredients in a high power blender and cover.

Blend on high for about 3 minutes, or until smooth.

Pour into tall glasses and serve right away.

Berry Mango Smoothie

Number of Servings: 2

You will need:

- 2 cups frozen mango chunks
- 2 cups frozen raspberries and/or blueberries
- 4 cups almond milk

How to Prepare:

Combine all the ingredients in a high power blender and cover.

Blend on high for about 3 minutes, or until smooth.

Pour into tall glasses and serve right away.

Green Tea and Raspberry Smoothie

Number of Servings: 2

You will need:

- 1 cup brewed green tea

- ½ cup frozen blueberries

- ½ cup halved seedless grapes

How to Prepare:

Combine all the ingredients in a high power blender and cover.

Blend on high for about 3 minutes, or until smooth.

Pour into tall glasses and serve right away.

Healing Ginger Smoothie

Number of Servings: 1

You will need:

- 2 ice cubes

- 2 fresh basil leaves

- 1 cup diced carrot

- 1 Tbsp peeled fresh ginger

- 1 Tbsp freshly squeezed lemon juice

How to Prepare:

Combine all ingredients in a high power blender and cover.

Blend on high for about 3 minutes, or until smooth.

Pour into tall glasses and serve right away.

Peppermint Fruit Smoothie

Number of Servings: 2

You will need:

- 1 cup peppermint tea

- ½ cup chopped fresh fennel

- 2 kiwis, peeled

- 2 apples, peeled, cored, and quartered

- 8 ice cubes

How to Prepare:

Combine all the ingredients in a high power blender and cover.

Blend on high for about 3 minutes, or until smooth.

Pour into tall glasses and serve right away.

Banana and Kale Energy Smoothie

Number of Servings: 2

You will need:

- 3 kale leaves, ribs and stems removed
- 1 large banana, peeled
- 5 dates, pitted
- 1 ½ cups hemp or almond milk
- 1 Tbsp vanilla protein powder

How to Prepare:

Combine all the ingredients in a high power blender and cover.

Blend on high for about 3 minutes, or until smooth.

Pour into tall glasses and serve right away.

Salad Recipes

Cucumber and Carrot Salad
Number of Servings: 6

You will need:

- 9 small organic carrots, peeled and sliced thinly
- 1 large cucumber, sliced thinly
- 2 fennel bulbs, sliced thinly
- 1 ½ cups chopped fresh parsley
- ¾ cup chopped fresh mint
- 1/3 cup freshly squeezed lemon juice
- 3 Tbsp extra virgin olive oil
- Sea salt and freshly ground black pepper, to taste

How to Prepare:

Place the carrot, cucumber, and fennel in a bowl, then toss well to combine. Add the mint and parsley, then toss again. Set aside.

In a bowl, combine the olive oil and lemon juice. Whisk vigorously until combined, then pour the mixture over the salad. Toss well to coat, then refrigerate for at least 30 minutes, or/ until chilled.

Best served chilled.

Roasted Beet and Quinoa Tabbouleh

Number of Servings: 3

You will need:

- 2 large garlic cloves, minced

- ½ lb beets

- 2 cups water2 cups fresh arugula

- 1 cup quinoa, rinsed thoroughly

- ½ cup pomegranate seeds

- ¼ cup cold-pressed olive oil

- 2 ½ Tbsp chopped fresh parsley

- 2 Tbsp freshly squeezed lemon juice

- 2 Tbsp chopped fresh mint

- 2 Tbsp chopped almonds

- ¼ tsp sea salt

How to Prepare:

Set the oven to 350 degrees F to preheat. Line a baking sheet with aluminum foil and set aside.

Poke the beets all over with a sharp knife or fork, then lay them on the prepared baking sheet. Bake for 30 to 45 minutes, or until tender. Transfer to a cooling rack and allow to cool. Meanwhile, boil the water in a pot over high flame and stir in the quinoa. Reduce to low flame, cover, and simmer for 15 minutes or until the quinoa has completely absorbed the water. Turn off the heat and set aside, covered.

Once the beets are cool enough to touch, peel off the skins then slice into bite-sized cubes. Place them in a salad bowl, then pour the lemon juice, and olive oil on top. Add the garlic, parsley, mint, and cooked quinoa, then mix well to combine.

Lay the arugula on a serving platter and heap the beet and quinoa mixture on top. Garnish with pomegranate seeds and serve right away.

Corn and Scallop Salad

Number of Servings: 3

You will need:

- ¾ lb scallops

- 3 corn cobs, boiled

- 1 large mango, peeled and diced

- 1 small avocado, peeled and diced

- 1 red bell pepper, seeded and diced

- 3 ½ cups mixed greens

- 2 Tbsp chopped fresh cilantro

- 2 Tbsp freshly squeezed lemon juice

- 2 Tbsp freshly squeezed lime juice
- 1 ½ Tbsp cold-pressed olive oil
- 1 ½ Tbsp seafood seasoning
- 1 lime, sliced into wedges

How to Prepare:

Season the scallops with the seafood seasoning, then set aside.

Place a skillet over medium high flame and heat through. Once hot, add the olive oil and swirl to coat. Add the scallops and cook for about 2 minutes per side, or until opaque. Transfer to a plate and set aside.

Scrape the kernels off the cooked corn cobs, then place in a bowl. Add the mango, avocado, and bell pepper. Pour in the juices and toss gently to coat.

Add the scallops to the mixture and toss gently to combine.

Lay the mixed greens on three plates, then heap the corn and scallop mixture on top. Garnish with cilantro and lime wedges, then serve right away.

Cranberry Fennel Salad

Number of Servings: 3

You will need:

- 3 cups baby arugula

- ¾ cup fresh cranberries (or any other berry in season)

- ¾ cup thinly sliced fennel

- 4 ½ Tbsp balsamic vinegar

- 3 Tbsp chopped almonds

- 1 ½ Tbsp chopped fresh mint

How to Prepare:

In a salad bowl, combine the baby arugula, cranberries, fennel, and mint. Toss well to combine.

Drizzle the balsamic vinegar over the salad, then toss again to coat. Sprinkle the almonds on top, then serve right away.

Spinach and Pea Salad with Feta

Number of Servings: 3

You will need:

- 3 cups baby spinach leaves

- 1 ½ cups fresh peas, or frozen and thawed

- ½ cup watercress

- ¼ cup fresh mint leaves

- 2 Tbsp olive oil

- 2 Tbsp cubed feta cheese

- 1 ½ Tbsp pumpkin seeds

- ¾ tsp creamed horseradish

- Sea salt and freshly ground black pepper , to taste

How to Prepare:

Pour the peas into a pot and add enough water to cover by about an inch. Cover and place over medium high flame.

Bring to a boil, then reduce to a simmer. Simmer for about 10 minutes or until the peas are tender. Drain thoroughly and set aside.

Place a small skillet over medium low flame and heat through. Once hot, stir in the pumpkin seeds for 3 minutes to toast, then transfer to a plate and set aside.

Combine the watercress, horseradish and olive oil in a food processor. Blend until combined, then season with salt and pepper to taste. Transfer to a bowl and set aside.

Combine the spinach, peas, mint, pumpkin seeds, and cubed feta in a mixing bowl. Divide into three servings, then pour the watercress dressing on top. Serve right away.

Avocado and Broccoli Salad

Number of Servings: 2

You will need:

- ½ lb broccoli, rinsed thoroughly

- 1 small ripe avocado

- 1 Tbsp cold-pressed olive oil

- 1 Tbsp freshly squeezed lemon juice

- ½ Tbsp Dijon mustard

How to Prepare:

Chop the broccoli into small, bite-sized pieces, then steam until crisp tender in a steamer pot or microwave. Set aside in a colander to cool completely.

In a small bowl, combine the olive oil, lemon juice, and Dijon mustard. Mix well, then set aside until ready to serve.

Right before serving, halve the avocado and discard the stone. Scoop out the flesh and slice into bite-sized chunks. Place in a bowl and add half the dressing. Toss well to coat.

Add the cooled steamed broccoli and then the remaining dressing. Toss well to coat, then serve right away.

Soup Recipes

Hearty Vegetable Lentil Soup
Number of Servings: 4

You will need:

- ¾ lb dried lentils
- 2 large carrots, peeled and chopped
- 1 celery stalk, chopped
- 1 onion, chopped
- 1 ½ cups crushed tomatoes, juices reserved
- 1 ½ Tbsp cold-pressed olive oil
- 1/3 tsp ground cumin
- 1 bay leaf
- Sea salt, to taste
- Freshly ground black pepper, to taste

How to Prepare:

Pour the lentils into a stock pot and add enough water to cover them by about 6 inches. Add the bay leaf, then cover and place over a high flame. Bring to a boil, then reduce to a simmer. Simmer for 25 to 30 minutes, or until the lentils are completely tender.

Add the cumin and onions into the pot of lentils, then stir in the celery and carrots. Simmer over medium low flame, loosely covered, for about 25 minutes.

Stir in the olive oil and tomatoes with their juices. Continue to cook until the soup becomes slightly thickened. Season to taste with salt and pepper, then ladle into soup bowls and serve right away.

Rice and Vegetable Soup

Number of Servings: 4

You will need:

- 1 small garlic clove, seeded and diced

- 2 small garlic cloves, minced

- 1 small red onion, minced

- 1 celery stalk, diced

- 1 small carrot, peeled and diced

- 4 cups vegetable or chicken broth

- 1 cup chopped kale

- 1 cup shredded cabbage

- ½ cup cooked brown rice

- ¼ cup chopped fresh parsley

- ¼ cup green lentils

- 1 Tbsp olive oil

- ½ tsp dried oregano

- Sea salt and freshly ground black pepper, to taste

How to Prepare:

Place a soup pot over medium flame and heat through. Once hot, add the oil and swirl to coat. And swirl to coat.

Stir in the onion until translucent, then add the garlic and sauté until fragrant. Add the bell pepper and carrot, then sauté until tender.

Stir in the cabbage and sauté until wilted. Add the lentils, oregano, and broth. Increase to high flame and bring to a boil. Once boiling, reduce to low flame and simmer for 30 minutes.

Add the parsley, kale, and brown rice, then stir and simmer for 10 minutes, or until the greens are wilted. Season to taste with salt and pepper, then serve right away.

Tilapia, Spinach and Leek Soup

Number of Servings: 3

You will need:

- 4 oz tilapia fillets, cubed

- 1 leek, sliced thinly

- 1 small garlic clove, minced

- 4 cups vegetable broth

- 1 ½ cups sliced fresh mushrooms

- 1 ½ cups fresh spinach leaves

- ¾ Tbsp seafood seasoning

- Canola oil spray

How to Prepare:

Pour the broth into a pot and bring to a boil over a high flame. Once boiling, stir in the leek, mushrooms, and garlic. Reduce to low flame and simmer for 10 minutes.

Meanwhile, lightly coat a skillet with canola oil and place over medium high flame.

Season the fillets with seafood seasoning, then place in the pan. Cook for 3 minutes per side, then transfer to the pot of soup. Simmer for 5 minutes, then stir in the spinach leaves. Turn off the heat and stir until the spinach is wilted.

Ladle into soup bowls and serve right away.

Sopa de Lima

Number of Servings: 6

You will need:

- 3 garlic cloves, minced
- 1 jalapeno pepper, seeded and minced
- 21 oz canned diced tomatoes
- 6 cups chicken or vegetable broth
- 2 ½ cups cooked diced chicken
- 1 ¼ cups chopped yellow onion
- 1/3 cup chopped fresh cilantro
- 4 ½ Tbsp freshly squeezed lime juice
- 1 ½ Tbsp olive oil
- ¾ tsp ground cumin
- 1/3 tsp dried oregano
- ¼ tsp black peppercorns
- Sea salt, to taste
- 1 lime, sliced into six wedges

How to Prepare:

Place a pot over a medium high flame and heat through. Once hot, add the oil and swirl to coat. Sauté the onion until translucent, then stir in the garlic and sauté for 1 minute or until fragrant.

Stir in the peppercorns, cumin, oregano, and allspice, then sauté until fragrant.

Pour in the broth, then bring to a boil. Stir in the tomatoes, chicken, minced jalapeno, and lime juice, then season to taste with salt.

Reduce to medium low flame and simmer for 10 minutes, then ladle into soup bowls and serve right away.

Roasted Apple and Butternut Squash Soup

Number of Servings: 3

You will need:

- 1 small butternut squash, peeled and chopped
- 1 baking apple, cored and quartered
- 1 large yellow onion, quartered
- 1 large garlic clove
- 3 cups vegetable broth
- 1 ½ Tbsp cold-pressed olive oil
- Sea salt, to taste
- Chili powder, to taste

How to Prepare:

Set the oven to 400 degrees F to preheat. Place the squash, onion, apple, and garlic in a roasting pan and add the olive oil on top. Toss well to coat, then season with salt and pepper.

Roast for 25 to 30 minutes, or until fork tender. Stir once every 10 minutes.

Once the apple and squash are tender, transfer half of them into a food processor. Add 1 ½ cups of vegetable broth, then blend until smooth. Pour into a soup pot, then add the remaining broth with the roasted apple and squash mixture.

Stir well over a medium flame until heated through and thoroughly combined. Adjust seasonings to taste, if needed.

Ladle into soup bowls, then serve right away.

Cashew Cauliflower Curry Soup

Number of Servings: 3

You will need:

- 1 small red onion, minced
- 1 small cauliflower, rinsed thoroughly
- 2 ½ cups coconut milk
- 1/3 cup water
- 2 ½ Tbsp chopped unsalted cashews
- 2 Tbsp chopped fresh cilantro
- 1 Tbsp curry powder
- 1 tsp cold-pressed olive oil
- ½ tsp raw honey
- ½ tsp ground turmeric
- 1/8 tsp ground cinnamon
- Sea salt, to taste

How to Prepare:

Pour the cashews into a food processor and blend until finely ground. Add the water and blend again until thoroughly combined. Pour into a bowl and set aside.

Place a small soup pot over a low flame and add the olive oil. Swirl to coat, then sauté the onions until translucent. Stir in the cauliflower and sauté until almost tender.

Add the cashew milk, coconut milk, honey, curry, turmeric, and cinnamon. Then, add more water to cover the solids, if needed. Cover and cook for about 10 minutes over low flame, or until the cauliflower is tender.

Turn off the heat, uncover, and allow to cool and thicken slightly. Then, blend the soup using an immersion blender or food processor until smooth.

Reheat over a low flame, then season to taste with salt. Ladle into soup bowls and serve right away.

Conclusion

I hope this book was able to help you treat or prevent chronic inflammation.

The next step is to develop the right habits that will prevent you from developing chronic inflammation for good. Aside from following the Anti-Inflammatory Diet, it will help if you exercise regularly in order to strengthen your body. It's also advised that you try not to get stressed out too much by incorporating relaxing strategies such as yoga or meditation into your everyday schedule.

Now that you have learned how you can be in charge, let all the knowledge you've gained help put your plan, towards eliminating chronic inflammation, into action. You alone are truly responsible for your health and wellbeing, so treat your mind and body with kindness. When you do, you will realize that you become naturally more productive and happy than you have ever been before.

Matthew Ward